Autistic Spectrum Disorder (ASD) Autism

A Complete Guide to Understanding an Autistic Person

Juanita E. McGrath

DISCLAIMER

Table of Contents

Introduction

Autism spectrum disorder, also known as ASD, is a developmental disability that is caused by differences in the brain. Patients diagnosed with ASD might have a recognizable difference, like a genetic condition. There may be other unknown causes. Scientists believe that ASD has multiple causes, and that these causes interact with one another to change typical patterns of human development. There is a great deal more that we do not yet know about these causes and how they influence individuals who have an autism spectrum disorder. Autism spectrum disorder (ASD) can cause people to behave, communicate, interact, and learn in unusual ways compared to most other people. The majority of the time, there is nothing about their appearance that sets them apart from other people. Ability levels can vary greatly among those who have an autism spectrum disorder (ASD).

For example, some individuals with autism spectrum disorder (ASD) may have advanced conversational skills, while others with the disorder may be nonverbal. Others with ASD are able to work and live independently with little to no assistance at all, while others with ASD require a great deal of assistance in their day-to-day activities.

ASD manifests itself typically before the age of three and may continue throughout a person's entire life, despite the fact that symptoms may become less severe as time passes. Early on in life, some children display symptoms of autism spectrum disorder (ASD). In some cases, the manifestation of symptoms might not take place until the child is at least 24 months old. Some children with autism spectrum disorder (ASD) learn new skills and meet developmental milestones until they are between 18 and 24 months old, at which point they either stop learning new skills or lose the skills they already had.

As children with autism spectrum disorder (ASD) mature into adolescents and young adults, they may have difficulty forming and maintaining friendships, communicating with peers and adults, and comprehending the behaviors that are expected of them at school or on the job. They may be brought to the attention of healthcare providers if they also have conditions such as anxiety, depression, or attention deficit/hyperactivity disorder, all of which are more common in people with autism spectrum disorders than in people without autism spectrum disorders.

Chapter one

To what exactly does the term "autism spectrum disorder" refer?

Autism spectrum disorder, also known as ASD, is a form of developmental disability that can result in severe difficulties in social interaction, communication, and behavior. People with ASD can have a wide range of symptoms, skill levels, and levels of disability. A "spectrum" includes all of these thingsSD

A developmental disability is one that has an impact throughout a person's life on their ability to communicate and interact socially with other people. One individual in every one hundred is diagnosed with autism, and there are approximately 700,000 autistic children and adults living in the United Kingdom.

Autism is a spectrum disorder that affects people differently. People who are autistic, just like everyone else, have their own unique set of advantages and disadvantages.

Who exactly is affected by ASD?

Autism is a spectrum disorder that can affect people of any race, ethnicity, or socioeconomic background. Boys are affected by this condition at a rate that is four times higher than girls. According to the Centers for Disease Control and Prevention (CDC), about one in every 54 children in the United States has an autism spectrum disorder (ASD).

Having autism

Simply having the diagnosis of autism does not mean that a person is sick or suffering from a disease. It indicates that your brain operates differently than the brains of other people.

It is a trait that you inherit from your parents. Autism symptoms could present themselves when a person is very young or much later in life.

If you have autism, you will always have the condition, regardless of how old you get.

Autism is not a disease that can be "treated" or "cured" by medical professionals. However, there are some individuals who require assistance with particular activities. You don't have to let the fact that you have autism stop you from leading a happy life.

People with autism are no different from anyone else in that they have strengths and weaknesses just like everyone else.

Being autistic does not prevent a person from having friends, developing romantic relationships, or finding gainful employment. Having said that, it is possible that you will need additional assistance in order to complete these tasks. Autism can be viewed as falling on a spectrum. This suggests that no two people with autism are exactly alike.

Some autistic people require little or no assistance. Others may need the daily assistance of a parent or other caregiver at all times. People with autism can range in IQ from low to extremely high. Some individuals with autism have intelligence levels that are average or even higher than average.

Some individuals with autism experience learning difficulties. This means that they might have trouble taking care of themselves and might need help doing day-to-day things.

People who have autism frequently have other medical conditions, including the following:
Attention deficit hyperactivity disorder (ADHD), dyslexia, sanity, depression, and epilepsy are some of the conditions that are associated with ADHD.

Chapter two

Manifestations of Autism

Autism's primary manifestations are difficulties in social communication and repetitive behaviors.

Behaviors that are constrained and performed repeatedly

Even if you don't notice them at first, symptoms can start in early childhood, last into adulthood, and make life hard.

Causes of Autism

There is not one specific cause that can be pinpointed for autism spectrum disorder. Because of the complexity of the disorder as well as the fact that the symptoms and severity can vary, it is highly likely that there are multiple causes. There is a possibility that genetic and environmental factors are both involved.

Genetic factors; Autism spectrum disorder is thought to be caused by a gene or gene combination that is inherited from both parents. A genetic disorder such as Rett syndrome or fragile X syndrome may be associated with autism spectrum disorder in certain children. This can be the case. Other children who have mutations in their genes may have an increased likelihood of developing autism spectrum disorder. It is possible that other genes have an effect on the development of the brain, how brain cells communicate with one another, or the severity of the symptoms. Some genetic changes seem to be passed down from one generation to the next, while others seem to be caused by random chance.

Environmental Factors: Scientists are looking into whether or not autism spectrum disorder can be caused by things like viral infections, medications, or problems that happen during pregnancy.

Autistic people face unique challenges.

1: **Difficulties with social interaction as well as communication.**

Interaction with other people

People with autism have difficulty understanding both verbal and nonverbal language, such as gestures and tone of voice, and this makes communication challenging for them. Some autistic people are unable to speak at all or have very limited speech, whereas other autistic people have excellent language skills but have difficulty understanding sarcasm or tone of voice. Other challenges include taking things literally and being unable to understand abstract concepts; needing additional time to process information or respond to questions; and repeating what other people say to them (this is called echolalia).

Communication with other people

People with autism often have difficulty "reading" other people, which means they have trouble recognizing or comprehending the emotions and motives of other people, as well as having difficulty expressing their own feelings. Because of this, navigating the social world can become extremely challenging. People who have autism might give the impression of not being caring.

Seek time alone when they feel overwhelmed by other people, don't look for comfort from other people, seem to act "weird" or in a way that isn't socially appropriate, and have trouble making friends.

2. Behaviors that are limiting and repetitive

People who are autistic may also engage in repetitive movements such as flapping their hands, rocking, or using an object repeatedly, such as twirling a pen or opening and closing a door. They may also have trouble with social interaction and communication. The majority of autistic people engage in these behaviors on a regular basis because they find them enjoyable. However, some autistic people do so because they find that doing so helps them relax when they are feeling anxious or stressed.

Alterations to a person's usual routine can also cause autistic people a great deal of distress and anxiety. It could be something as simple as a bus detour that causes them anxiety.

It could also be the adjustment to major events like Christmas or changing schools. It could also be dealing with uncertainty at work.

3, **Either an overabundance or a deficiency in sensitivity to light, taste, sound, and touch.**

People with autism can have heightened or decreased sensitivity to a variety of stimuli, including sounds, touch, tastes, smells, light, colors, temperatures, and pain. For instance, they might find certain ambient noises, like the music playing in a restaurant, to be intolerably loud or distracting, whereas other people are able to tune them out or ignore them altogether. This can lead to feelings of anxiety as well as physical distress. As a result of the discomfort it causes them, many autistic people choose not to hug, which can be misunderstood as being distant and uncaring.

Many autistic people steer clear of everyday settings because of the sensitivity issues they struggle with. Particularly stressful and overwhelming in terms of sensory stimulation can be environments such as schools, workplaces, and shopping malls. There are many straightforward adjustments that can be made in order to make environments more accessible to people with autism.

4: **Hobbies or interests with a narrow focus**

Many autistic children have intense and narrowly focused interests in a specific topic at a young age. These may change over time or remain unchanged permanently. Autistic people have the potential to excel in their areas of interest and enjoy the satisfaction of passing on their knowledge to others. Trains are an example that conforms to the stereotype, but they are just one of many. Greta Thunberg, for instance, feels very strongly about the need to safeguard the environment.

People with autism, like everyone else, get a lot of pleasure from doing things they find interesting, and they see these activities as essential to their happiness.

Many autistic people have an advantage at work and in school because they can focus very hard on tasks. However, they run the risk of becoming so focused on one topic or activity that they forget about other things in their lives.

5: Unbearable levels of anxiety

Anxiety is a common problem for autistic adults, particularly in social settings or when they are forced to adapt to new circumstances. It is possible for it to have an effect on a person's mental and physical health, as well as a detrimental effect on the standard of living of autistic people and their families.

It is essential for autistic people to develop coping mechanisms to help them deal with the anxiety they experience and learn to identify the triggers that bring on their symptoms. However, a significant number of autistic people have difficulty identifying and controlling their feelings. More than one-third of people who have autism suffer from serious mental health problems, and far too many autistic people are not succeeding in life.

6: Meltdowns and total shutdown

A person with autism may have a meltdown or withdraw completely when they feel overwhelmed by the demands placed on them. These are trying experiences that leave one exhausted.

A person is said to have a meltdown and temporarily lose behavioral control when they are completely overcome by the circumstances in which they find themselves. This loss of control may manifest itself verbally (for example, yelling, screaming, or crying), physically (for example, kicking, lashing out, or biting), or in both ways at the same time.

Children's meltdowns are frequently misunderstood as tantrums, and parents and their autistic children frequently face hurtful comments and judgmental stares from members of the public who are less understanding.

A shutdown may seem like a less severe problem to those who are looking in from the outside, but it can be just as crippling. The act of shutting down, also known as "switching off," is a response that people have when they feel overwhelmed. "Just as frustrating as a meltdown," said one autistic woman, "because of not being able to figure out how to react how I want to, or not being able to react at all; there isn't any 'figuring out' because the mind feels like it is past the point of being able to interpret." A "shutdown" is when an autistic person is unable to respond to stimuli in any way.

How to Communicate with an Autistic Person and Its Implications.

1: **Getting and keeping their attention is essential.**

Always address the person by their name so they know you are speaking to them specifically.

Make sure that they are paying attention before you proceed to ask them a question or give them an instruction. When someone is paying attention, different people will pick up on different cues that indicate this.

2: **Use their interests and hobbies, or the activity they are doing at the moment, to get their attention.**

The processing of information

When a person with autism is trying to process information, it can be challenging for them to ignore irrelevant details. The condition known as "overload," in which no more information can be processed, can occur when there is an excessive amount of information. To be of assistance, I will speak more slowly and less frequently.

3: Make use of specific key words and emphasize and repeat them throughout your writing.

Give the other person time to think about what you've said and formulate a response by pausing between each word and phrase you say to them.

Try not to ask an excessive number of questions.

Cut down on the amount of nonverbal communication you use (e.g. eye contact, facial expressions, gestures, body language).

4: Create the impression that you could care less.

Look for time alone when they feel overwhelmed by other people, don't seek comfort from other people, seem to act "weird" or in a way that isn't socially appropriate, and have trouble making friends.

Limiting and repetitive patterns of behavior

People who have autism may also engage in repetitive movements such as flapping their hands, rocking, or using an object repeatedly, such as twirling a pen or opening and closing a door. They may also engage in ritualistic behaviors such as grooming and washing their hands repeatedly. They might also have difficulty communicating and interacting socially with others. However, some autistic people engage in these behaviors on a regular basis because they find that doing so helps them relax when they are feeling anxious or stressed. The vast majority of autistic people engage in these behaviors on a regular basis because they find them enjoyable. However, some autistic people engage in these behaviors because they find that doing so helps them enjoy themselves when they are under stress or anxiety.

Alterations to a person's typical routine can cause autistic people a great deal of distress and anxiety, as the same goes for neurotypical people. It could be something as innocuous as a detour taken by the bus that gives them cause for concern. It could also be the adjustment to significant life events, such as moving schools or celebrating Christmas for the first time. It could also be dealing with ambiguity in one's professional life, either an abundance or a lack of sensitivity to light, taste, sound, and touch, respectively.

People who have autism can either have an increased or decreased sensitivity to a variety of stimuli, including sounds, touch, tastes, smells, light, colors, temperatures, and pain. For instance, they may discover that particular background noises, such as the music that is playing in a restaurant, are intolerably loud or distracting, whereas other people are able to tune them out or ignore them entirely. Because of this, one may experience feelings of anxiety in addition to physical discomfort. There are many autistic people who choose not to hug because it makes them feel uncomfortable. However, this behavior can be misinterpreted as being distant and uncaring.

Because of the difficulties they have processing sensory information, many autistic people avoid environments that are typically part of their daily lives. Environments such as schools, workplaces, and shopping malls can be particularly stressful and overwhelming in terms of the amount of sensory stimulation they provide. Many simple changes can make it much easier for people with autism to get around in their environments.

Activities or interests that can be categorized according to a particular subfield

A significant number of autistic people, even when they are young, have intense and highly concentrated interests in a particular subject. It's possible that these will shift over time, or they might stay the same forever. Autistic people have the potential to excel in their areas of interest and enjoy the satisfaction of passing on their knowledge to others. People with autism have the potential to excel in their areas of interest. Trains are just one example of something that fits the stereotype, but there are a lot of other examples as well. Greta Thunberg is one person who has a deep-seated conviction that there is an urgent need to protect the environment.

People who are autistic, just like everyone else, get a great deal of pleasure out of participating in pursuits that they find interesting, and they believe that engaging in these activities is necessary to their happiness.

Many autistic people have an advantage in the workplace and in school because of their ability to concentrate intensely on tasks. However, they run the risk of becoming so preoccupied with one topic or activity that they neglect other aspects of their lives. This can be a problem for autistic people who have jobs or who are in school.

Levels of anxiety that are intolerable.

Adults who have autism often struggle with anxiety, particularly in social situations or when they are required to adapt to new circumstances. It is possible for it to have an effect on a person's mental and physical health, as well as a negative effect on the standard of living of autistic people and their families. Also, it could hurt the quality of life of the people who take care of autistic people.

It is essential for autistic people to develop coping mechanisms to help them deal with the anxiety they experience and learn to identify the triggers that bring on their symptoms. In addition, it is important for autistic people to learn to identify the triggers that bring on their symptoms. On the other hand, a sizeable percentage of autistic people struggle to recognize and manage the emotions that they experience. More than one-third of people who have autism also suffer from serious mental health problems, and far too many people with autism are not succeeding in life.

Power outages and total meltdowns:

When a person with autism feels overwhelmed by the demands that are placed on them, they may completely withdraw from social interaction or have a meltdown. These are challenging experiences that can leave one feeling completely spent.

When a person is completely overpowered by the circumstances in which they find themselves, we say that they have a meltdown and temporarily lose behavioral control. Meltdowns can also be caused by a temporary loss of inhibition. This loss of control may manifest itself verbally (for example, yelling, screaming, or crying), physically (for example, kicking, lashing out, or biting), or in both of these ways at the same time. Children's meltdowns are frequently misunderstood as tantrums, and parents and their autistic children frequently face hurtful comments and judgmental stares from members of the public who are less understanding. Meltdowns in children are a common symptom of autism spectrum disorder.

Those who are looking in from the outside may have the impression that a shutdown is a less severe problem than it actually is, but it can be just as crippling. People have a tendency to "switch off," which is another term for the act of shutting down, when they experience feelings of being overburdened. "Just as frustrating as a meltdown," said one autistic woman, "because of not being able to figure out how to react how I want to, or not being able to react at all; there isn't any 'figuring out' because the mind feels like it is past the point of being able to interpret." "Just as frustrating as a meltdown," a "shutdown" is when an autistic person can't respond in any way to stimuli.

The Challenges of Communicating with Autistic Individuals and Their Implications

It is essential to get their attention and continue to keep it.

Always use the person's name when addressing them so that they understand that you are speaking to them in particular.

Before you proceed to ask them a question or give them an instruction, you should check to see if they are paying attention first. Different people will pick up on different cues that indicate someone is paying attention.

To get them interested, you should use their interests, hobbies, and the activity they are already doing.

The operation of processing information

It may be difficult for a person with autism to ignore unimportant particulars when they are trying to process information because of the way their brain works. When there is an excessive amount of information, the condition known as "overload," which occurs when no more information can be processed, can take place. This can happen when there is a lot of data. To help:

Sight

UNDER-SENSITIVE

Objects take on a very dark appearance or lose some of their distinguishing characteristics.

The vision in the center is hazy, but it is relatively clear on the edges.

Attention is drawn to the object in the middle of the frame, and details on the edges become less clear.

This person is clumsy, can't tell where things are in space, and has trouble throwing and catching.

OVER-SENSITIVE

Vision that is distorted, making it appear as though objects and bright lights are moving around.

Images may fragment.

Focusing on one part of something is much easier and more enjoyable than looking at the whole thing.

Because they are sensitive to light, they have trouble falling asleep.

You could make adjustments to the environment, such as lowering the amount of fluorescent lighting, providing sunglasses, installing blackout curtains, and/or constructing a workstation in the classroom. A workstation is a space or desk that has high walls or divides on both sides to block out visual distractions.

Sound

Under-sensitive

- Speak more slowly and not as frequently in order to be of assistance to them.

- Make use of specific terms that serve as key words, and be sure to emphasize and repeat those terms throughout your writing.

- By pausing between each word and phrase that you say to another person, you give them the opportunity to reflect on what you've just said and come up with a response.

- Make an effort to limit the number of questions that you ask.

- Reduce the amount of nonverbal communication you use in your interactions with others (e.g. eye contact, facial expressions, gestures, body language).

OVER-SENSITIVE

It is possible for noise to become amplified, and for sounds to become distorted and muddled.

They may be able to pick up on conversations taking place further away.

If you can't block out sounds, especially background noise, it's hard to focus on a task.

You could be of assistance by:

Close doors and windows to lessen the impact of noise from the outside.

preparing the individual prior to going to places that will be noisy or crowded

We offered earplugs as well as music for people to listen to.

Setting up a workstation with a screen in the classroom or office and moving the person so they are not near any doors or windows.

Smell

UNDER-SENSITIVE

Some people don't have a sense of smell and can't smell strong smells, which can include their own body odor.

Some people have the habit of licking objects in order to get a better understanding of what they are.

You could help by getting into a routine of frequently washing your hands and using strong-smelling products to take people's minds off of things that shouldn't be there, like feces, that smell strongly.

OVER-SENSITIVE

- It's possible for odors to be overwhelming and potent. This may cause problems with urination and defecation.

- He dislikes people who choose to wear distinctive fragrances, including shampoos, perfumes, and the like.

You can make a difference by avoiding the use of perfume and scented cleaning products, shampoos, and detergents, and by ensuring that the surrounding environment is as fragrance-free as possible.

Taste

Under- sensitive

A person with under sensitive taste enjoys foods that are spicy, consumes or chews on non-edible items such as feces, stones, dirt, soil, and grass, as well as metal and other metals.

The term for this condition is *pica*.

OVER-SENSITIVE

Because of the extreme sensitivity of his taste buds, he finds that certain flavors and foods are far too powerful and overwhelming for his palate. has a restricted eating plan.

Because of the discomfort that can be caused by certain textures, you are only allowed to consume smooth foods like mashed potatoes or ice cream.

Some people with autism may prefer foods with a lack of flavor or have a craving for foods with a strong flavor. As long as there is some variety in a person's diet, this is not necessarily a cause for concern.

Touch

UNDER-SENSITIVE(Insufficiency of sensitivity to contact)

A person who holds others tightly must first do so themselves before they can be said to be applying pressure to others. Demonstrates a high capacity for bearing pain.

It's possible that they won't be able to feel any food in your mouth.

They could injure myself.

They take great pleasure in having heavy things piled on top of them, such as weighted blankets.

Smearing feces on his face because he enjoys the way it feels.

They chew on anything they can get into their mouth on, including things that aren't edible and clothing.

You might be of assistance if you:

- You should offer smearing options that have similar textures, like jelly or cornstarch mixed with water.
- Providing chewable alternatives to latex, such as tubes, straws, or hard candies (chill in the fridge).

OVER-SENSITIVE

People may dislike being touched, which can have an effect on their relationships with other people. Touch can be painful and uncomfortable. People may dislike being touched.

They have a strong aversion to having anything resting on their hands or feet.

challenges with brushing and washing the hair.

 It's possible that you won't like the texture of many foods.

Only certain articles of clothing or surface textures are acceptable to them. One thing you could do to help is to make sure that you approach people from the front whenever you are going to touch them.

Keep in mind that a hug, despite its intended purpose, can actually cause discomfort.

transforming the consistency of food in some way, such as by puréeing it.

You can help by:

- By slowly putting different things in the person's mouth, like a flannel, a toothbrush, and different foods, the person can get used to the different feelings.

- Gradually expose the child to a variety of tactile experiences, such as making a collection of materials available in a box.

- Including allowing a person to do things on their own (like brushing their hair and washing their hair), so that they can do what they want to do; removing any tags or labels from clothing; turning clothing inside out so that there are no seams; and allowing a person to do things on their own.

This gives the person the freedom to wear clothes that fit their own level of comfort.

BALANCE(vestibular)
UNDER-SENSITIVE

The need to rock, swing, or spin in order to receive sensory input

You could spread awareness about activities that are beneficial to the growth of the vestibular system. This could mean doing things like rocking horses, swings, roundabouts, seesaws, catching a ball, or practicing climbing steps or curbs in a smooth way.

OVER-SENSITIVE

- We struggle with activities like sports that require us to control our movements, such as throwing a ball or hitting a ball.
- When participating in an activity, it can be challenging to come to a full stop as quickly as possible.
- Automobile sickness
- When performing tasks that require one's head to be tilted backwards or one's feet to be lifted off the ground, there are bound to be complications.

You can help by breaking down tasks into smaller, more manageable steps and using visual reminders like a finish line.

Body awareness (also known as proprioception) is the process by which our bodies provide us with information about where we are in space and how each of our body parts is moving.

UNDER-SENSITIVE

- They stands too close to other people because they are unable to judge personal space and accurately measure their distance from other people.
- Finds it challenging to maneuver through rooms and sidestep obstructions.
- May have interactions with people around them.

You might be of assistance if you:

- Placing pieces of furniture around the room's edge in order to make it easier to move around in it.

- Deep pressure can be applied through the use of weighted blankets.

- Utilizing different colored tape to demarcate boundaries and the "arm's-length rule" to determine personal space, which involves maintaining a distance of at least one arm's length from other people.

OVER-SENSITIVE

- Difficulties with fine motor skills, such as those required for manipulating small objects like buttons or shoe laces

- When they want to look at something, they move their whole body.

You could be of assistance by supplying 'fine motor' activities like lacing boards and the like.

Synaesthesia

Synaesthesia is an extremely uncommon condition that may be present in autistic individuals. An experience can enter one sensory system and leave the body through a different system. As a direct consequence of this, a person may listen to a sound but interpret it as a hue instead. To put it another way, the color blue will become audible to them.

Therapy and equipment

We can't make suggestions about how effective specific therapies, interventions, or pieces of equipment are.

Music therapists use a wide range of musical instruments and sounds to help their patients develop their senses, most often their hearing.

Occupational therapists make plans for their patients and often make changes to the environment to help their clients with sensory differences live as independently as possible.

Speech and language therapists often use sensory stimuli, which can help in many ways, such as encouraging and supporting the development of language and interaction.

Some people believe that colored filters can be helpful, despite the fact that there is very little research evidence to support this hypothesis.

Although autism itself is not a mental illness, autistic people, like everyone else, can have both good and poor mental health.

Autism is characterized by a high incidence of meltdowns. Meltdowns in autism are not the same thing as temper tantrums, despite what the general public believes, but they are frequently confused for one another. Figure out how to predict, recognize, and cut down on the number of episodes of meltdown that your family member or the person you support has.

Just what is meant by the term "meltdown"?

A severe reaction to an overwhelming circumstance is referred to as a meltdown. It takes place when a person is completely overcome by the circumstances they are in at the moment and loses control of their behavior as a result. This loss of control may show itself verbally (for example, yelling, screaming, or crying), physically (for example, kicking, lashing out, or biting), or both.

The term "meltdown" should not be confused with "temper tantrum." It is not a manner that would be considered impolite or improper. It is easy to understand why someone would have a meltdown when they are completely overwhelmed and their condition makes it difficult for them to express themselves in any other way.

A person with autism can show how frustrated they are in many different ways besides having a meltdown.

They might also withdraw from situations that they find challenging and refuse to interact with other people.

What action should I take?

If someone is having a breakdown or isn't responding to you, it's best not to pass judgment on them. A person who is autistic and the people who care for them can benefit tremendously from it.

Give them some space and time to get over the amount of information or feelings that is too much.

You should ask them (or their parent or friend) in a calm manner if they are okay, but you should keep in mind that it may take them longer to respond than you might anticipate.

Make room—do your best to create a quiet, safe environment. You should ask people to move along and not stare; turn off the loud music; and dim the lights. In fact, you should try anything you can think of to reduce the amount of information that is being provided.

Chapter three

The screening process and the diagnosis

Because there is no reliable medical test, such as a blood test, for diagnosing autism spectrum disorder (ASD), the condition is notoriously difficult to identify. The behavior of the child as well as the child's developmental history are looked at by doctors when making a diagnosis.

Asperger's syndrome (ASD) can be diagnosed as early as 18 months of age. The diagnosis provided by an experienced professional can be regarded as reliable once the patient reaches the age of two [1]. However, a definitive diagnosis is not provided to a great number of children until they are much older. There are some individuals who do not get a diagnosis until they are in their teenage years or even later. Because of this delay, people with autism spectrum disorders might not get the help they need as soon as they need it.

Children with autism spectrum disorder need to be diagnosed as soon as possible so they can get the services and help they need.

for the purpose of helping them realize their full potential This process is broken down into a few distinct steps.

Keeping an Eye on the Development

Monitoring a child's development is an ongoing, active process that involves keeping track of a child's progress and encouraging parents and childcare providers to have conversations about the child's current knowledge, skills, and capacities. Developmental monitoring includes watching your child grow and seeing if they meet the typical developmental milestones, or skills that most children achieve by a certain age, in areas such as playing, learning, speaking, behaving, and moving.Keeping an eye on your child's development means watching them grow and seeing if they reach the normal developmental milestones.

Parents, grandparents, teachers who work with young children, and other caregivers can all keep an eye on a child's growth and development.

To gauge how well your child is doing in each stage of development, you can use a simple checklist like the one given here. If you've noticed that your child isn't meeting certain developmental milestones, you should talk to your child's primary care doctor or nurse about your concerns and ask what could be wrong and how to fix it.

An Evaluation of the Status of Development

The screening for developmental delays looks at how well your child is growing and developing.

The process of developmental screening is one that is carried out in a more formal setting than the monitoring of developmental progress. It is a standard procedure that is done at some well-child checkups, no matter if there is anything to worry about or not.

During routine well-child visits, the American Academy of Pediatrics (AAP) recommends performing developmental and behavioral screenings on all children of these ages:

- Over a period of nine months.
- Duration of 18 months duration of 30 months.

Also, the American Academy of Pediatrics (AAP) recommends that all children be tested for autism spectrum disorder (ASD) during regular well-child visits when they reach these ages of 8 months and 12 months.

The screening questionnaires and checklists that are used are founded on research that compares your child to other children of the same age.

The ability to communicate, move, and think, in addition to one's behaviors and feelings, may be evaluated. The screening process for developmental delays can be carried out by a physician or nurse, in addition to other professionals working in healthcare, the community, or schools. It's possible that your physician will ask you to fill out a questionnaire as part of the screening process. Screening should be performed at an earlier or later age than the ages that are recommended if you or your doctor have any concerns about it. If a child is at a high risk for autism spectrum disorder (ASD; for example, having a sibling or other family member with ASD) or demonstrates behaviors that are sometimes associated with ASD, then additional screening should be performed on the child. You have the right to ask your child's healthcare provider to do developmental screening tests on your child more often if they don't already.

Developmental Diagnosis

A brief screening tool test does not provide a diagnosis, but it can indicate whether or not a child is on the right developmental path or whether or not a specialist should be consulted. A diagnosis of development is not provided by the test. If the screening tool identifies a potential area of concern, it is possible that a formal evaluation of the child's development will be necessary. This formal evaluation is a more in-depth examination of a child's development than the informal evaluation, and it is typically performed by a trained specialist such as a developmental pediatrician, child psychologist, speech-language pathologist, occupational therapist, or any other specialist. The specialist may interview the child's parents or caregivers, question the child, give the child a structured test, observe the child, or have the parents and caregivers fill out questionnaires. With the help of the results of this formal evaluation, which show both the child's strengths and weaknesses, you will be better able to plan for his or her future.

Asperger syndrome is an umbrella term for a group of conditions that were previously classified as separate illnesses: autism disorder, pervasive developmental disorder not otherwise specified (PDD-NOS), and Asperger syndrome. The diagnostic procedure is something that you should be able to comprehend, and your doctor or another healthcare provider can help you with that.

An official developmental evaluation is the way to go if you want to know for sure whether or not your child needs early intervention services. In certain situations, the specialist may suggest that your child go through genetic counseling and testing.

Chapter four

Treatment

The goals of the various treatments currently available for autism spectrum disorder (ASD) are to alleviate symptoms that get in the way of daily functioning and reduce overall quality of life. People who have autism spectrum disorder each have their own distinct set of advantages and disadvantages, as well as treatment requirements that are particular to their condition. Nevertheless, there are a variety of treatments available that can help reduce symptoms and improve functional abilities. People with autism spectrum disorder (ASD) have the best chance of using all of their skills and abilities to the fullest when they get the right therapies and interventions.

The treatments and interventions that are most successful are frequently individualized for the specific patient. However, the majority of people who have ASD respond best to interventions that are highly structured and specialized. Treatment can assist individuals with autism with day-to-day activities and, in some cases, reduce symptoms of the condition. Because of this, treatment plans are usually made by a team of professionals, are based on working together, and are different for each patient.

Treatments are able to be administered in a variety of environments, including educational, health, community, and home environments, or in any combination of these settings. To ensure that treatment goals and progress are met, it is essential for providers to communicate with one another, as well as with the person who has autism spectrum disorder (ASD) and their families.

Additional services can help people with autism spectrum disorder (ASD) improve their health and day-to-day functioning as well as facilitate their participation in social and community activities as they enter adulthood and graduate from high school. Some people might need help to finish school, get a job, find a place to live, or get to work.

Different Methods of Treatment

There is a wide variety of treatment modalities to choose from. Even though some treatments use more than one method, these treatments can generally be put into the following groups:

Methods Based on Behavior

The goal of behavioral approaches is to alter behaviors by gaining a better understanding of what comes before and after the behavior in question. The majority of the evidence suggests that behavioral approaches are the most effective way to treat ASD symptoms. As a result of their widespread acceptance among teachers and medical professionals, they are now utilized in a variety of schools and treatment clinics across the country. People diagnosed with ASD are often given the well-known behavioral treatment of Applied Behavior Analysis (ABA) (ABA). The goal of ABA is to improve a wide range of skills by reinforcing the behaviors that are desired and discouraging the behaviors that are not desired. The progress being made is being measured and monitored.

Two of the teaching strategies used in ABA are known as Discrete Trial Training (DTT) and Pivotal Response Training (PRT) (PRT).

Developmental Approaches

Instructions are provided on a sequential basis in DTT, which is used to teach a desired behavior or response. Lessons are simplified down to their elemental building blocks, and the responses and behaviors that are desired are praised and rewarded. Ignorance is given to responses and behaviors that are not wanted.

Personal Responsibility Training

The PRT procedure is carried out outside of a medical facility rather than inside of one. The purpose of the Personal Responsibility Training (PRT) is to assist individuals in the development of a select group of "pivotal skills" that can serve as a foundation for the acquisition of a wide variety of additional competencies. One example of an important skill is the ability to start a conversation with other people.

Developmental Approaches

The primary focus of developmental approaches is either the enhancement of particular developmental skills, such as language or physical abilities, or on a wider range of developmental abilities that are interconnected with one another. Combining behavioral approaches with developmental approaches is something that is done frequently.

People who have autism spectrum disorders typically participate in speech and language therapy as their primary forms of developmental treatment. Individuals can benefit from speech and language therapy by increasing both their understanding of and their ability to use speech and language. Some individuals diagnosed with ASD are able to communicate verbally. Others may talk using signs, gestures, pictures, or devices that make electronic communication easier.

Patients undergoing occupational therapy are taught skills that enable an individual to live as independently as possible. Putting on clothes, eating, taking a bath, and interacting with other people are all examples of skills. In addition to these services, occupational therapy may also include the following:

One of the goals of sensory integration therapy is to help people respond better to sensory input that is either too limited or too much.

Improvements in motor skills, whether they be minute finger movements or larger trunk and body movements, are one of the goals of physical therapy. The Early Start Denver Model (ESDM) is a comprehensive method for child development that is founded on the principles of applied behavior analysis. It is recommended for use with children ranging in age from 12 to 48 months.

Parents and therapists use play, social exchanges, and shared attention to help children improve their language skills, social skills, and learning abilities in natural settings.

Methodologies for Educational Practices

Educational therapies are typically delivered in a group setting, such as a classroom. One type of educational approach is known as the Treatment and Education of Autistic and Related Communication-

Handicapped Children (TEACCH) approach. The theory that underpins TEACCH is that individuals with autism can benefit from a curriculum that emphasizes continuity and visual learning. It provides educators with strategies that can be used to modify the structure of the classroom in order to improve academic and other outcomes. For example, a person could write down or draw their daily activities and then put them in a prominent place.

Methods that Consider Social Connections

Treatments that focus on improving social skills and emotional connections are known as social-relational therapies. In certain social-relational approaches, the use of parents or peers as mentors is encouraged.

The Floor Time model, which is also called the Developmental, Individual Differences, and Relationship-Based model, tells parents and therapists to focus on the person's interests to help them talk more.

The Relationship Development Intervention (RDI) model is built around activities that make people more motivated, interested, and able to have shared social interactions.

"Social stories" are straightforward descriptions of what to expect in a social situation.

People with autism spectrum disorder (ASD) can benefit from social skills groups because they give them a structured place to practice social skills.

Techniques Used in Pharmacology

There is currently no medication that can effectively treat the primary symptoms of autism spectrum disorder (ASD). There are medications that treat co-occurring symptoms, which can improve a person's functioning even if they have an autism spectrum disorder (ASD). Medication, for instance, may be helpful in the management of excessive energy, inability to focus, or self-harming behavior such as banging one's head or biting one's hands, among other examples. Medication can also assist in the management of co-occurring psychological conditions such as anxiety or depression, in addition to medical conditions such as seizures, sleep problems, or stomach or other gastrointestinal issues. This can be beneficial for patients who have both conditions.

It is essential to have a discussion about the possibility of using medication with a medical professional who has prior experience treating patients diagnosed with autism spectrum disorder (ASD). This is the case with both medications that require a prescription and those that can be purchased without one.

People, their families, and their doctors need to work together to keep track of how the condition is progressing and how the body is responding to the treatment in order to ensure that the adverse effects of the medication do not outweigh its positive effects.

Psychological Methods

People with ASD can benefit from psychological treatments for a variety of mental health concerns, including anxiety, depression, and other conditions. Cognitive-behavioral therapy, also known as CBT, is a method of psychological treatment that places an emphasis on gaining an understanding of the connections that exist between one's thoughts, feelings, and actions. During cognitive behavioral therapy (CBT), the individual and the therapist work together to identify goals, and then the individual changes how they think about a situation in order to change how they react to that situation.

Therapies for alternative and complementary medicine

Certain individuals, including parents, opt for treatments that do not fit into any of the aforementioned categories. These forms of treatment are collectively referred to as complementary and alternative therapies. Treatments that are considered alternative and complementary are frequently used in conjunction with methods that are considered more conventional. Some examples of alternative therapies include mindfulness and relaxation training, special diets, herbal supplements, animal therapy, arts therapy, chiropractic care, and mindfulness meditation. Before starting any kind of complementary or alternative treatment, people and families should always talk to their main doctor.

Conclusion

This book's objective is to provide readers with an understanding of the significance of interacting with autistic children and adults, as well as the difficulties associated with doing so. This book discusses the factors that make communication and engagement difficult, as well as the ways in which people with autism engage, the impact of sensory differences on communication and engagement, the impact of the environment on communication and engagement, the rules of engagement, and how to engage.

As a result of this activity, participants gain a better understanding that challenging autism behavior is rarely straightforward or the result of a single cause. The impact of autism, sensory processing, quality of life, and the roles that professionals and families play are all topics that are covered in this guide.

It educates participants about the sensory experiences that people with autism go through as well as how to provide support in a practical manner. This guide provides information on how people with autism are affected by differences in their senses; how to differentiate between hypersensitivity, hyposensitivity, and synaesthesia; and practical strategies that can be used to support people in their daily lives at home and in the workplace.

9 79835 37 65400